The Weight Agency Method

by Bobbie Piety

Excel Your Way To Weight Loss Success!

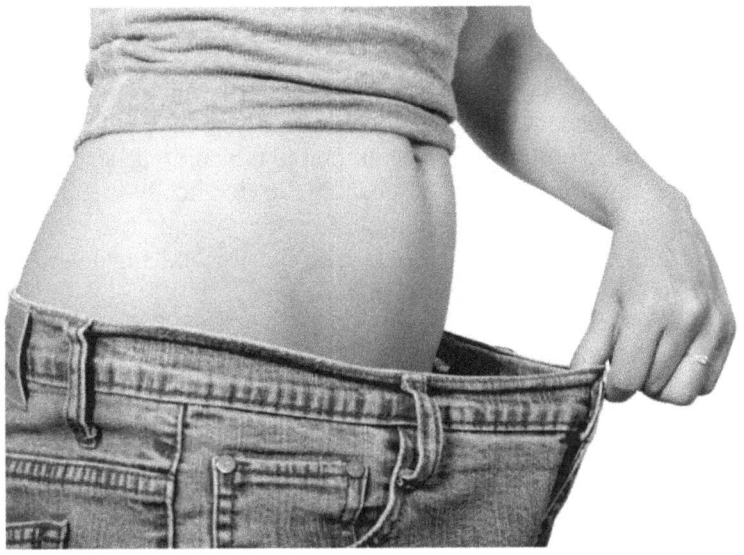

How you got fat

How to lose the fat

How to keep the fat off

The **last book** you will ever need on losing weight!

The Weight Agency Method

by Bobbie Piety

Excel Your Way to Weight-Loss Success!

How you got fat
How to lose the fat
How to keep the fat off

This is the **last book** you will ever need on losing weight and is a companion to a Microsoft Excel® spreadsheet for tracking progress. It is short and to the point, appealing to the no-nonsense person—especially the technically-oriented person who likes a scientific, foolproof weight loss plan tailored to his or her own tastes. This method empowers YOU to regain control over YOUR weight!

Table of Contents

1. Introduction

If you are looking for an easy way to lose weight, there isn't one. If you are not prepared to do what you have been avoiding, and are just looking for easy answers, put this booklet down—it is not for you. If you are bored with numbers and not willing to weigh your food and record your calories, protein, carbohydrates, and weight daily, this is not for you. But, after a lifetime struggle with weight and trying almost every diet ever invented, I have finally found something that truly works and I will share it with you. It ain't easy! But, I can tell you how to make it as easy as possible, how to lose a LOT of weight as safely as possible, how to make it fun, and how to keep excess fat off. I will also explain how you got fat and why, and what to watch out for in the future, which will help keep it off and keep you healthy. The recording of calories eaten takes less than 5 minutes per day and will show you the EXACT consequences of what you eat!

Increasingly, we work less physical work and more work while sitting down. The days of physical labor on a farm, or of trekking through woods to hunt and gather food, before machines changed agriculture, are largely gone. Now, we sit in offices, drive vehicles instead of walking, and sit down to watch television after dinner. At the same time, food scientists put great effort into making food appealing to us in novel ways. They layer fat, salt, and sugar in the right proportions, with the right flavorings and spices, not only to make us eat more, but also to make us eat when we are no longer hungry. They make food tasty and fun to eat, so we eat more and become addicted to the blood sugar highs that result. Have you ever wondered why fast-food restaurants all seem to use the same, ultra-white, fluffy, sweet buns for their burgers instead of offering whole-wheat alternatives? Or "season" their fries with additional starch? Yes, food releases the same neurotransmitters in the brain that are released when a heroin addict gets his opiate fix, or that a smoker gets from a cigarette. This neurotransmitter release is the body and brain's reward system and is necessary for the survival of a species. Suppose you woke up tomorrow and no food tasted good and did not release this reward to the brain. Why would people bother eating at all, let alone go to great lengths to hunt, gather, or cultivate food? Our very survival mechanisms cause us to eat more than we should, and modern life not only eliminates the necessity for expending great energy to acquire it, but also provides an abundance of calorie-laden, tasty foods. The big question is, *why isn't everyone overweight*? The answer is that a vast number of us *are* overweight, even if we are not considered obese.

This book will explain all this in detail and arm you with what is necessary to lose extra weight and keep it off. It is a companion to a Microsoft Excel® spreadsheet that will help you track your progress and see if you are on track for meeting a specific weight loss goal. The spreadsheet will also show you what adjustments you need to make to keep making the progress you want. More importantly, it will educate you as to what foods have what nutritional complement, enabling you to make educated choices in what you eat. This book also tends to "cut to the chase" and spares the reader of many details of the metabolic process. For those people who wish to study those topics in detail, the online Wikipedia® (http://www.wikipedia.org/) is an excellent reference to further research the details contained herein. The USDA nutritional database also is an important web site for looking up the nutritional content of foods that we eat: (http://www.nal.usda.gov/fnic/foodcomp/search/).

I will also not list copious references but I will occasionally embed a source—usually from the Internet—as I did above. Nowadays, the Internet offers an incredible wealth of information (and misinformation) so I will leave it to the readers to focus on aspects mentioned in this booklet that particularly interest them. Much of my research has come from the Internet and numerous books that I have read. I have followed everything from the infamous Cabbage-Soup Diet to the effective, but difficult to follow, Carbohydrate Addict Diet (http://www.carbohydrateaddicts.com/), as well as almost every diet I could find. None worked very well for me, frankly, though most had great ideas. And this is the reason why I have written the last book you will need on weight loss.

If it is not apparent from the above, you will need a computer with Microsoft Office® (or equivalent) and Internet access to get maximum benefit from this book.

Disclaimer: As with all diets and eating plans, you should consult with your doctor before undertaking the suggestions contained in this book.

Note: Microsoft Office® and Microsoft Excel® are registered trademarks of the Microsoft Corporation. Wikipedia® is the trademark of the Wikipedia, the Free Encyclopedia.

2. How We Got Fat

We ate too much. End of chapter. It would be the end of the chapter if we did not peel the onion a bit to find out *why* we ate too much. Eating an <u>extra</u> apple a day will not necessarily "keep the doctor away," but eating that extra apple daily will add about 12 pounds per year in stored fat. Do that for ten years and WOW—what happened? We would find ourselves hugely obese—all from an extra apple a day. That extra apple adds about 120 calories to one's intake. Since there are 3500 calories to a pound of fat, simple math helps us to realize that this extra eating adds a pound of weight per month, or 12 pounds per year. Many overweight people do not eat a horrendously large amount of food, but merely the equivalent of an <u>extra</u> apple a day. I see slim people often eating far more than I would dare, but it is clear that their metabolism is higher than mine and/or they are more active. For many people, however, eating even a small amount of extra food each day will add many pounds over months and years.

A lot of us eat eat much more than an extra apple a day. We enjoy fattening snacks, pizza or burgers for lunch, perhaps a nice steak, potato, wine, and dessert in the evening. This is often much more than the 120 extra calories that the extra apple provides. In fact, if you "want fries with that," that alone can add 500 calories to an already calorie-laden meal.

A good friend, Bea, is an executive in a high-tech company. She travels frequently, eats in restaurants most of the time, and loves wine. Being busy and always on the go, she does not have time to "diet," so she eats what looks good on the menu and accompanies her dinner with at least two glasses of wine, which add more than 300 daily calories to her full diet. She is about 60 or 70 pounds overweight!

Another friend, Dana, is always dieting and tries to work it off at the gym. She is a very emotional woman and frequently gets upset or angry. When something upsets Dana, she cheers herself up with a sugary treat. She loves bread and eats it at most meals. Dana is about 75 pounds overweight.

Wanda is a very active friend who is always on the go but eats lunch in restaurants almost daily. She thinks salads are diet food and Caesar salads are her favorite, not realizing that they often contain more calories than a cheeseburger. Wanda drinks diet cola a lot and when she does not eat a salad, she often has a cheeseburger and fries. Wanda is about 75 pounds overweight.

Frank likes to snack a little each evening but is otherwise "good." This snacking, little by little, has put about 40 extra pounds on him, despite the fact that he eats prudent meals ordinarily. Frank likes bread with meals and this helps cycle his blood sugar and appetite.

These friends are typical of the many people who struggle with weight in our modern society. To some extent, active people burn off the abundant calories in typical diets, and our bodies try to maintain our weight by increasing our Basal Metabolic Rates (BMR) that compensate for part of our extra food intake. We may sense our clothes feeling tighter. We may go to the gym to burn off some of the fat or "diet," which usually means feeling "starved." If you had a large order of French fries with your lunch, you would have to do <u>vigorous</u> aerobics for an *hour* to burn those extra fries off. Now, I don't know about you, but I would be an exhausted puddle of perspiration if I exercised vigorously for an hour, if I could even maintain it for that long. Given the choice, I would rather forego the fries than to sweat for an hour, but maybe that is because I am fat. Yes, I am FAT. I have been fat all my life and have become an expert at *getting* fat, but my research has finally enabled me to understand all the reasons why I am fat, and I am sharing those reasons with you. I am losing my fat as I write this book.

The Calories3 spreadsheet that I wrote to track my food intake, weight, and results assures me that I will be 50 pounds lighter by November 2011 (I started this effort in mid-July). And, I can assure you, in writing, that I will be slim by this time next year, 120 pounds lighter than I was a month ago. How is *that* for confidence? I have the confidence because all the information I have accumulated has come together in this booklet, spreadsheet, and eating suggestions. I say "suggestions" because I am explaining the consequences of your food choices and letting you choose what to eat and what to do. The spreadsheet does not lie and if you are not getting the results you want, you will know *exactly* why.

I do not like exercise! I do not like to perspire. I would rather drive somewhere than walk. I would rather watch a TV or movie than go jogging or even walking most of the time. I suspect that you are much like this too, because you are reading this book. As an overweight person, I can tell you that exercise is a *lot* of work! With every step I take, I am carrying an extra 120 pounds! That's huge! Imagine trying to play tennis, take a walk or ride a bike, or do much of anything physical with a sack of concrete (90 lbs. plus) strapped to your back. That would be a total drag! That was a LOT of work, which makes me hungry. So, I'll sit down and eat some pizza instead. Or, I could "diet" with some cabbage soup, but accompany my meal with 500 calories of bread. And so it goes. We have let ourselves eat that extra apple a day or we have indulged in that order of fries once a week, or we had a pizza on Sunday, and so on, little by little, until we got fat. And, as we got fat, exercise became more difficult, so we did less, compounding the problem. Being "good" all week, then splurging on a Saturday pizza—with all else unchanged—will add 10-15 pounds a year! And, most of us do this sort of chaotic eating year in and year out, resulting in gaining *many* pounds over the years.

People tell us "just eat less," not realizing that we often eat less than they (the skinny ones) do. We go on diets and avoid the fattening foods. We eat modestly. But, exercise is difficult when one is fat and sweating is no fun. Not only that, but fat is a good insulator. I joke that I have "built-in R-19 insulation." So, as I exercise even a little, I overheat and perspire a lot. Again, no fun. Also, with that insulation that I carry, my Basal Metabolic Rate (BMR) drops and I burn fewer calories, *further* compounding the problem. Starvation diets lower the BMR too, thus exacerbating the problem even more. Losing weight seems impossible. We can maintain our weight or gain weight when eating "normally". We see slim people eating burgers, drinking milkshakes, enjoying pizza, enjoying fancy desserts, and we get depressed—why can't *we* eat such things and be slim? And, with this depressed feeling, some of us—like Dana—eat a snack for the neurotransmitter release in our brains. We need our fix.

Many of us have become accustomed to the usual portions provided by restaurants. When McDonald's first introduced the Quarter Pounder®* forty years ago, it was considered a BIG burger. Now, most fast food restaurants in 2011 offer 1/3lb or 1/2 lb burgers, including McDonald's. What happened? We have slowly become accustomed to larger portions. What used to be a large burger is now the norm, and a large burger now is *twice* the size of the one 4 decades ago. Almost all restaurants offer larger portions nowadays because they do not want their customers going home hungry or telling their friends how they got "ripped off" at So and So's restaurant. Besides, along with larger portions come larger prices, so everyone wins.... except the person unwittingly *getting trained to* consume increasing amounts of food.

Some people successfully combat this by asking for a to-go box when their waiter brings them their food, and they put half of it in the box to take home before even beginning their meals. But, frankly, although I sometimes do this, I seem to forget too often, or I am too hungry from letting my blood sugar cycle, so I do not bother. Not many people do. So, we eat more. Couple that habit with what some of our parents taught us about finishing what was on our plates when we were children and you now know how we got to where we are—overweight, if not downright fat or, heaven-forbid, obese.

*Quarter Pounder® is a registered trademark of McDonald's Corporation.

3. Food Addiction

When we think of addicts, we think of heroin addicts injecting drugs into their veins or crack smokers or speed users. Or, we think of smokers who have difficulty stopping tobacco use, or alcoholics who spend their days drunk and addicted to alcohol. But, many of us are *food addicts*! The drug and alcohol users all get a neurotransmitter release in their brains when they indulge in their drug of choice, but the food addict gets that *same release* when enjoying fattening foods! The more the calories, the greater the fix: A deep-fried onion, a cheeseburger dripping with melted cheese perhaps with bacon added, a basket of fries, a milkshake with added chocolaty goodies, pizza with extra cheese and tasty toppings, and so on. We get our fix when we eat those foods, similar to the high that drug users get from their drug fix.

What happens when the drug addicts do not get their fixes? They crave them. The drug addicts become obsessed with getting their next fixes to avoid painful withdrawal. What happens when food addicts do not get their fixes? They get hungry… then famished—they are experiencing *their* withdrawal. They, too, crave their next fix, but they call it being hungry or "starved." If we do not get our food fix, our stomachs growl and cause discomfort. This is withdrawal! We become focused on getting some food to satisfy the hunger and ease the discomfort… and waiting to get our next fix.

Tell a smoker to "just chew some gum," instead of having a cigarette, and they will likely laugh at you. Gum is not what they want or need. Gum does not provide the fix. Similarly, when well-meaning friends tell the food addict "just eat a carrot or some celery," the addict feels like stuffing that in them, because it does absolutely nothing for the addict's yearning—there is no fix—which is the fat/sugar/salt fix food addicts need to satisfy their hunger… their fix.

Since food is so necessary for life, and we need the vitamins and nutrition from vegetables, fruits, and proteins, why does that carrot or celery not satisfy us? Why do we want pizza or a burger or fries or sweets instead? The reason for this is two-fold. First, we have become used to these "goodies" in life— the calorie-laden tasty, crunchy, salty, fatty, sweet foods that dominate much of the prepared foods we find in grocery stores and restaurants. Food scientists know that these are the foods we like and they provide them for us in abundance. Have you ever noticed how the produce and meat/fish/dairy aisle in a supermarket comprise a small percentage of the store? Yet, the areas containing snacks, cookies, sweetened cereals, bakery goods, and other prepared foods tend to dominate. They do not have coolers with steaks or produce in the checkout aisles. Instead, they have candy and chips for our impulse buys. In a way, the food industry has helped turn us into food addicts. Biology did the rest and we let ourselves be duped into helping.

Laying blame on the food industry is somewhat misguided because if you were a food manufacturer, you would want people to like your product and buy it, which is quite reasonable. Similarly, if you ran a restaurant, you would want your customers coming back. So, little by little, with the aid of taste tests, food manufacturers have discovered what we like, what we keep buying, and what dishes we order when we keep returning to our favorite restaurants. These same food manufacturers have discovered that they can increase the amount of sugar in a product by adding salt—or vice versa. They can take a salty product and add sugar and that modified food may no longer taste too salty. Too sweet? Add some salt. Add fat and you can increase the salt and sugar even more. It is this salt/fat/sugar combination that is found in almost all snack foods—foods that we like and which we buy more. Not only is salt, sugar, and fat an easy and inexpensive way to add weight to a product that is sold by weight, but also the additives induce us to eat more of it, to buy more of it, and to order more of it in restaurants. And then there is flour; think of all the tasty treats made from flour. Most of these tasty treats contain quite a bit of salt, sugar, and fat along with the flour. All these "goodies" are loaded with calories, provide a spike in our blood sugar, jolt a subsequent neurotransmitter release in our brains, and help make us become food addicts.

4. Glycemic Index

What happens in our bodies when we eat carbohydrates? Basically, our blood sugar begins to rise, triggering the pancreas to produce insulin. This also occurs to a lesser extent with fats, but carbohydrates are more easily digestible so they induce a greater insulin response. Insulin regulates carbohydrate and fat metabolism by causing our tissues to take glucose from the blood and store it in the liver and muscles as glycogen. Insulin also stops the body from burning fat for energy and instead switches to the readily available glycogen. Glucose in the bloodstream can become toxic if the insulin is not available to remove it from the bloodstream and store it as glycogen. This is what happens to diabetics who lack insulin: poor circulation to the extremities can result in amputation from gangrene, and lack of circulation to the eyes can cause blindness.

When the blood glucose levels drop, the body begins to use fat as an energy source through glycogenolysis by using stored fats in our bodies and converting them to ketones, which are then used for energy. <u>The important thing to note is that if there is an abundance of glucose in our diet, and therefore plenty of glycogen, our stored fat will **not** be used for energy because the glycogen is a more easily used source of energy.</u>

We don't drink glucose, so where does it come from? Glucose comes mostly from sugars and starches that we eat, as well as fats. The digestive details are beyond the scope of this book, but the carbohydrates (sugars, starches) that we eat are ultimately converted to glucose for use by the cells. Excess glucose is converted to fat and stored in our fat cells. Fats are metabolized into ketones and converted to energy by the cells. Table sugar—sucrose—is a mix of glucose and fructose. There are other sugars like lactose, maltose, dextrose, and other simple sugars that come from various foods we eat.

How quickly our bodies convert carbohydrates to glucose is a function of a food's *glycemic index*. Foods high in glycemic index are quickly broken down and converted to glucose. Those foods low in glycemic index take more time to digest and are slow to be converted to glucose. Fruits, vegetables, legumes, whole grains, nuts are usually low glycemic index foods. Refined grains, white bread, white rice, rice cakes, breakfast cereals, starchy vegetables, and table sugar are usually high glycemic index foods.

Overweight people often indulge in high glycemic index foods and, when doing so, set off an interesting chain of events that is <u>exceptionally important to understand</u> if you wish to understand how you gained excess weight, what to do to lose it, and how to keep it from coming back. Due to habitually eating such foods, our bodies become insensitive to insulin, and more and more insulin is required for proper functioning due to heavy carbohydrate overload. The pancreas can eventually "burn out" and fail to produce sufficient insulin, which results in type 2 diabetes. This can lead to complications from high blood sugar that include increased risk of heart attacks, strokes, kidney failure, amputation of limbs, and even blindness and deafness. In other words, extreme cycling of blood sugar is something to be avoided, yet food addicts often continue until it is too late.

Michel Montignac (http://www.montignac.com/) discusses glycemic index and its effects on diet and offers a useful table of glycemic indices: http://www.montignac.com/en/ig_tableau.php. Refined snack foods are near the top of this table, while greens, vegetables, nuts, and seeds are near the bottom. Beware that low glycemic index does not imply low calories. Oil has pure calories but also has a low glycemic index, for example; and

14

rice cakes may be low in calories but are very high in glycemic index. Another useful glycemic index table can be seen at: http://www.glycemicindex.com/ and yet another at http://www.glycemicindex.ca/glycemicindexfoods.pdf. Amazingly, dates, boiled potatoes, and several other common foods elicit a higher insulin response from the body than glucose itself and should be avoided by people wishing to lose weight. It should be noted, however, that consuming small amounts of these foods along with large amounts of *low* glycemic index, fibrous foods, can slow their absorption and lower their aggregate insulin response.

When people routinely eat large, fatty, high glycemic index meals, interesting physiological events occur. The Pavlovian response by the mind *anticipates* another typical meal and the body begins producing copious amounts of insulin even before it is necessary. This results in an initial drop in blood sugar, making us actually feel hungrier *even after we have begun eating*. We often eat faster to compensate and wind up overeating and feeling stuffed. Fat people with bulging waistlines—as opposed to those with small waists and large hips—often become this way by frequent overeating and stretching their stomachs.

The following graph shows a normal (or pre-diabetic) blood sugar response to high glycemic-index diets. The blue curve shows how the blood sugar initially drops a bit when a person begins eating, due to excess insulin being released by the pancreas, in anticipation of a calorie-laden, high carbohydrate meal. This drop in blood sugar then makes us eat ravenously and quickly. Our blood sugar begins to rise after we have already eaten too much and are bloated as a result, stretching our stomachs and intestines. Blood sugar rises quickly and we get our "fix." Then, after every calorie is wrung out and stored as fat, our blood sugar plummets as early as 3 hours later, making us feel hungry, then shortly later, "starved", and we overeat again, repeating the cycle. Contrast this with the red curve which shows the blood sugar after a person eats a low glycemic-index meal (after re-conditioning his or her eating habits). Blood sugar does not spike, but rises moderately and then falls very gradually. As the blood sugar falls, we metabolize stored fat to some extent. The slowly falling blood sugar means we get hungry later and if we do not eat right away, we are only slightly hungrier hours later. This is the desired eating habit to lose and maintain weight.

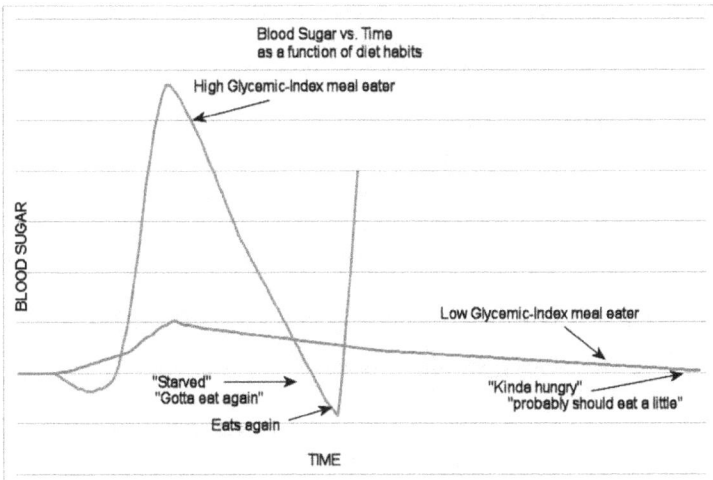

What puts "salt in the wound" of the above high-glycemic meal blue curve is that this eating pattern causes an over-abundance of insulin to be produced that does several things:

- It gives food addicts their fix—their "rush" from the rapid rise in blood sugar.
- It causes excess energy to be stored in cells.
- It causes fat already in cells to stay there.
- It causes a subsequent rapid drop in blood sugar, making us famished again.

16

After eating a fast-food cheeseburger and fries—which I knew had more than half the calories I needed in an entire day—I used to wonder why I felt extraordinarily hungry a few hours later, and absolutely famished if I didn't eat within an hour of the onset of hunger. It did not make sense; now it does. The typical fast food meal has a very high overall glycemic index, and is purposely so because it satisfies our food fix and causes us to come back for more… and to buy more because we are "starved." High glycemic-index foods literally addict some of us! This is great for the fast food industry, but not so good for fat people wanting to lose weight.

You have surely heard of the various diets that tout low carbohydrate intake. By keeping carbohydrates to a minimum—or consuming low glycemic index foods—the wild blood sugar swings are tamed, as shown in the red curve above. Blood sugar falls very gradually, augmented by the use of stored fat to a small degree. We get hungry eventually, of course, but it is not the intense, growling hunger experienced by the food addict in need of a fix. Instead of feeling famished soon after we notice the onset of hunger, the low glycemic index eating results in a *gradual* increase in hunger. I can be hungry at 5PM, and if the situation precludes me from eating until much later, I am only slightly hungrier by 7PM, and not even "famished" by 9PM. For this reason, I recommend watching the glycemic index of what we eat, even after we have achieved our weight loss goals.

Have you ever heard someone tell you "just eat some raw veggies when you're hungry"? Or an apple? You wonder what is wrong with that person. A carrot or apple *does not even begin* to satisfy the hunger that the food addict feels. No, addicts want a burger or pizza or a steak and potato, and so on—something that will "stick to our ribs" (literally). Raw veggies or an apple to satisfy hunger is a joke—it does virtually nothing for us and, in fact, may actually lower our

17

blood sugar initially, and make us feel hungrier as our Pavlovian insulin response over-produces the amount of insulin needed. Here is the good news. Within a week or two of following a low glycemic-index eating plan, you will have reconditioned your body to actually feel satisfied from fruit or vegetable snacks when hungry. You will have tamed your body's insulin response and will be well on your way to establishing "normal" eating habits and normal weight. You will still be able to have an occasional high caloric, high glycemic index meal, but that kind of meal must be the *exception* rather than the rule. I have found that if I indulge once per week or less, I can "get away with it." That is, my body will remain re-trained for low insulin response. Just as the Pavlovian response to frequent over-eating occurs, the reverse also occurs. It is as though the body is asleep when that occasional indulgent meal comes in and the excess is passed through instead of every last calorie being wrung out and absorbed.

5. How to Break the Cycle

Some people like to make changes to their lifestyles gradually, while others achieve success cold-turkey. I am of the cold-turkey camp, preferring to tough it out while my willpower is high and while my motivation is high. For me to gradually wean myself off of eating is akin to a smoker gradually trying to cut back—it is slow torture and erodes my will and leaves me discouraged. So, I am going to suggest to you that you follow my method, make your changes beginning tomorrow, and tough it out. You will be over much of the craving to eat your "contraband" within a week, and over most of the cravings within 2 weeks. I say "much" and "most" because if a person is hungry and sees deep fried onion rings, a bacon cheeseburger, and a chocolate milkshake, he or she will find this appealing. But, you will easily be able to resist it. Just like a drug addict out of rehab knows that they cannot have even one fix, the person following this diet will also realize the consequences of that one splurge. How many times have we done the "just once" and lied to ourselves, only to give up our dreams of being slim and eating healthily? Do not go down that road—it just is not worth it. But, do not fret—this is not forever. Once you acclimate your body to sensible eating, you can *occasionally* indulge in such foods. But, you may also find much of their appeal is gone, especially if you educate yourself as to what happens to your body when you eat foods containing partially hydrogenated fats. These contain *trans-fats* and cause inflammation of your arteries, leading to strokes, high blood pressure, and heart attacks. Sadly, most deep fried restaurant and commercially-prepared foods use partially hydrogenated fats. Nutritional scientists will tell you that NO amount of trans-fat is harmless to your body! If a "serving" contains less than half a gram of trans-fat, food manufacturers are allowed to claim "NO TRANS-FAT," but that is misleading. It is best to avoid any food with hydrogenated (partially or fully) oils, and be exceptionally wary of deep-fried restaurant foods.

We can change our bad eating habits not only to lose weight, but also to eat better quality foods and avoid the damage to our arteries that comes from high glycemic-index foods and trans- fats. To eat healthier and to be satisfied with less food, we can learn the appetite effects and calorie-to-nutrition impacts and nutritional content of the foods we eat.

Here is where the Calories3 spreadsheet comes in to help. We will use it to enter some basic parameters such as our starting date, our height, weight, our goal weight and goal date. The latter two entries will depend on your physician's advice. For me, I have set a *very* aggressive 50-pound goal in 18 weeks. That is about the maximum rate that anyone can lose weight and remain healthy. Of course, water weight comes off first in large numbers. One can lose a pound per day for the first 2 weeks, but this is not sustainable. Ultimately, I plan to lose 120 pounds, but the first 50 pounds is an intermediate goal. I will unwaveringly continue until I get all 120 pounds of fat off of me, and I will keep it off. My dear dad once proclaimed, "We spend half our lives ruining our bodies, then the other half trying to undo the damage". Truer words have not been spoken, and I am definitely well into my second half of my life. I've already used my "Get Out Of Jail" card and must lose the fat if I hope to achieve healthy living in this second half. I have gotten away, so far, without diabetes, without a heart attack, and without most of the maladies that can accompany a lifetime of being overweight. I do not want to push my luck; neither should YOU!

Essentially, we need to keep our carbohydrate intake low to avoid the wild blood sugar swings which leave us tired and hungry, and especially avoid the high glycemic index foods. The lower our carbohydrates are, the more our bodies rely on burning fat for energy to keep us going. However, vegetables and fruits contain numerous vitamins, minerals, fiber, antioxidants, and various other compounds necessary for good health, so I do not recommend a diet entirely devoid of carbohydrates.

When you suddenly switch from the eating patterns that made you and kept you fat, to an eating pattern that helps you lose weight, your body will scream bloody murder for a few days! You will feel hungry—starved, famished. You could eat a horse. But, recognize this as part of the withdrawal process and tough it out. You will get over it in a few days of prudent eating and will be well over the worst of it in a week's time, and almost completely over it in two weeks. Breaking this carbohydrate addiction is key to the success of this and most other diets.

The body takes a few days to undergo the chemical changes in which it becomes more efficient in burning stored fat for energy, but the body will definitely burn the stored fat if we optimize the conditions to let it do so instead of burning carbohydrates all the time.

Amazingly, you too will find that eating 300-400 grams of raw vegetables or an apple will keep your energy level up and your hunger down, all for a very low calorie impact. I used to eat 230 calorie energy bars during a round of golf, one of my passions, but now I bring a plastic bag with a couple of carrots to munch on in case I am hungry or notice that my coordination is dropping from low blood sugar. Much of the time, I do not even think of eating them, but I do if my teammates stop for food and I am reminded. I used to hate the people who said, "Oh, I forgot to eat lunch," and wondered what planet they were from. "Bitches!" I could not *fathom* not eating. Now, I understand it and am occasionally guilty of forgetting to eat too.

I can eat a **pound** of carrots and they only add up to 160 calories! Or a <u>pound</u> of zucchini is less than 100 calories. A <u>pound</u> of celery is 75 calories, and so on. On the other hand, an 8-ounce bag of potato chips contains <u>more than 1200 calories</u>!

Skipping meals is not good to do, however, because eating smaller meals and snacking (on low-calorie, healthy snacks) will keep one's blood sugar at a more even keel. But we do what our schedules allow and our appetites dictate. One acquaintance lost 75 lbs, swearing that she ate the same food as before, but dividing them into 6 meals instead of 2 or 3. And, it has been said that the Sumo wrestlers are fattened by starving them all day, then letting them eat anything they want at dinner time, which causes wide swings in their blood sugar, makes them overeat, and makes their bodies store almost every calorie eaten. That is how important it is to stop the wild blood sugar swings! Stopping these swings will take much effort for a week or two, but you will be delighted that you did stop and you will be amazed at how satisfied you will feel from much smaller amounts of food and lower glycemic index foods that would not even *begin* to satisfy your appetite before.

6. Basic Nutrition

It is important to eat a balanced diet from all the food groups—meat, fish, and dairy for protein, vegetables and fruit for vitamins, minerals, and fiber; and plenty of water to wash salts and metabolites from the body. That's WATER, not diet sodas or juices. Remember the Pavlovian response I mentioned earlier? Our bodies respond to diet sodas much the same way as if they were regular sodas, producing a dose of insulin to store the sugar. But, there is no sugar in the diet soda, so the insulin takes residual blood sugar and sequesters it in the liver and muscles, resulting in a blood sugar drop. Guess what that does? It makes us hungry. Scientific research has found that diet colas, which contain phosphoric acid and/or citric acid, leach calcium from our bones. The research said that while larger-boned men can get away with drinking colas to some extent, women will have detectable bone loss from drinking as little as one cola (diet or regular) per day. In short, drink ordinary water—it helps flush toxins from our bodies and provides some minerals. Incidentally, drinking distilled or de-ionized water will also leach calcium from our bones. Just drink tap water, which is usually as good as any bottled water, if not better, is less expensive and has less impact on the environment.

Important to note is that the more severe the calorie reduction, the more difficult it is to get sufficient nutrients required for healthy bodies and minds. An acquaintance went on a three-month extreme diet of only the canned diet shakes that can be found in most grocery stores and pharmacies. His choice resulted in a seizure which required hospitalization due to an electrolyte imbalance that caused permanent brain damage; he now requires ongoing medication. He lost 50 pounds but suffered greatly from hunger because these canned diet drinks are high in carbohydrates and cause the hunger-inducing blood sugar swings. So, avoid such extremes. In my opinion, less than 1000 calories per day is asking for trouble. For myself, I have chosen between 1100 and 1200 calories per day and, to date, am averaging 1204 at the time of this writing. I am also targeting my protein intake to be more than 100 grams per day. Experts say we should have 0.8g protein for every kilogram of body weight. To keep appetite under control, I am also trying to keep my carbohydrates relatively low, about 150 grams per day, and of course, I am avoiding the high glycemic-index ones. I do eat an occasional potato or piece of bread, but I keep this to an absolute minimum. When eaten with meat and other proteins, these high glycemic index foods are digested more slowly, reducing their impact on blood sugar. Because of such occasional splurges, my carbohydrate intake varies quite a bit, but the Calories3 spreadsheet tells me that I have been averaging under 150 grams per day.

Alcohol is another thing to minimize because it contains calories. A cup of wine contains about 160 calories and a cocktail can contain significantly more. Alcohol is metabolized before fat, slowing fat metabolization. It also relaxes muscles, somewhat, and reduces inhibition, both of which can lead to increased eating. While not a big deal, in my opinion, just know that it is not difficult to consume several hundred calories worth of alcoholic beverages in a social setting.

I used to enjoy a breakfast sandwich in the morning, which consisted of a toasted bagel, a fried egg, three thin slices of deli ham, and a slice of cheese. Then, I realized that the bagel—not only made of white flour and high in glycemic index—added 250 calories to my meal! Wow! That is almost ¼ of my daily allotment, and *doubles* the calories in the breakfast sandwich, not to mention what it does to my blood sugar and appetite a few hours later. Now, instead, I have two eggs, the same amount of ham, and the same amount of cheese for a total of 330 calories instead of 580 calories. I usually have a small bowl of fruit which adds 100 calories, to which I add the whey protein powder for another 130 calories, for the 32 additional grams of protein. So, my breakfast, when I eat the eggs, totals 615 calories—slightly more than half my daily quota—but provides 75 grams of protein. On other days, I may eat more fruit and add 175 grams of cottage cheese instead of the ham, eggs, and cheese, for 500 calories and 65 grams of protein. Today, I had 400 grams of fruit— that's *almost a pound*—and 200 grams of 2% cottage cheese and the whey protein for a 530 calorie breakfast. Contrary to my advice, I sometimes skip lunch or just snack on carrots, because I can do this without causing excessive hunger at dinner time. But that works for me. You may choose a different breakfast, but be very careful with cereals and breads as they contain many calories and spike the blood sugar. Occasionally, on a cold day, I will have a bowl of oatmeal, but I notice that its high carbohydrate content makes me hungry sooner. On days when I am more physically active, I may have 400 grams of carrots (almost a pound!) which is only 150 calories, and so on. I adjust my quantity of food and the type of food according to my daily quota and always try to eat a variety of foods to help assure getting a variety of vitamins and minerals. Some days, I find that I have only eaten 900 calories so I "splurge" a bit and have a 200-calorie snack, which might be fresh cherries, other fruit, or even some celery with a small amount of peanut butter. A bowl of berries with a tablespoon of ice cream makes a surprisingly delicious, yet low-calorie dessert. Even then, I avoid the high glycemic index foods or I will wake hungry and want to eat more. I cannot stress the importance of low glycemic index foods enough! Keep your blood sugar at an even keel and your appetite will remain under control, making it easy to stick to a calorie-deprived diet.

Not all proteins are the same. There are seven essential amino acids that the body requires and if one is missing, the body cannot use the others. Gelatin is almost pure protein but is far from complete, so gelatin is not a good dietary source of protein. However, <u>whey protein isolate is a complete protein</u> and I usually add a 35g scoop of it to one of my meals each day. The whey protein isolate provides 32g protein at a "cost" of 130 calories. The body digests the whey protein more slowly than a carbohydrate-only meal, and gives a full feeling for a longer time. Fat is also digested more slowly than carbohydrates and is one of the reasons that a completely fat-free diet is not recommended. Not only do our brains and bodies require some fat, but also a modest amount of fat will give us more satiety. I do <u>not</u> recommend fat-free foods; <u>low</u>-fat is much more prudent and effective.

The last thing I want to mention here is that one's calorie needs depend on one's weight and physical activity. If I am sedentary and my body's Basal Metabolic Rate slows down— and it will when I am reducing in weight—the caloric needs will also go down. So, you may find yourself starting out with 1500 calories per day, but later find that you must reduce this to 1200 as your weight drops further, to maintain the same rate of weight loss. The Calories3 spreadsheet lets you track this and allows you to make necessary adjustments to your food intake and energy output. Again, be VERY careful about dropping too low in daily calorie consumption because acquiring the proper nutrition becomes increasingly difficult and is risky. Always consult with your physician before going on any extreme diets.

7. Calories In, Calories Out

I have been talking mostly about what we eat and how to reduce calories consumed. As you know, our activities expend calories. A lumberjack or physical laborer can eat 4000 calories per day or more because he works hard all day and burns up his calories. But, if a small woman with an office job and a sedentary life tried that, she would quickly become huge. So, one way to increase your daily calorie allotment is to burn more calories through exercise—the dreaded E-word for many of us.

But, exercise does not have to be a sweaty, agonizing workout that is excruciating for a fat person who may be carrying the equivalent of a sack of concrete on their back in terms of excess weight. Also, to exercise away a donut or cheeseburger takes a LOT more exercise than it took to consume it. A cheeseburger contains 500-800 calories, on average, and according to http://www.nutristrategy.com/activitylist4.htm, it takes an hour of vigorous aerobics or running, or two hours of walking briskly, to burn that much energy. Is that cheeseburger or donut worth it? I think not. Frankly, I could not run or do aerobics for an hour, and I would be hard pressed to walk briskly for two hours. So, eating a burger and then working it off just isn't going to happen in my life, and not in likely yours. So, my choice—and likely yours—is to avoid the donut or burger in the first place.

But, having said that, I have to tell you that there *are* other ways to burn calories, though none are as dramatic as extreme aerobic strenuous exercise. Simply by walking a block or two to the store and back, or taking a stroll around your neighborhood, is something that most people *can* do, and that will burn maybe 100 calories or so. That deficit can help you lose weight more quickly, or can allow you to eat a bit more if that is what you choose to do. My point is that *any* physical activity is better than none, and any exercise you can get yourself to do will help increase your calorie output, not to mention usually making you more fit.

You can park in the furthest corner of the store parking lot when shopping, for example, or carry things by hand that you might otherwise put in your car. For me, walking is my most compatible form of exercise. Walking is not very aerobic unless I walk briskly, but it helps keep my legs strong and it does burn calories. And, remember too that I am carrying more than a sack of concrete worth of fat on my body, so this *is* indeed exercise. Standing burns roughly twice the calories that sitting does. Doing your own housework or gardening also burns more calories than paying a housekeeper or gardener. And, I do not mean that you must fire your hired help, if you have any, but there is no law that says that you cannot also do cleaning and gardening too. If you find ways to be active, even a little bit, you will burn more calories than just by sitting on your butt.

Building muscles is another way to burn more calories. Muscles burn calories not only when you are exercising to build them, but also when at rest, while you sleep. The more muscle mass you have, the more calories you will burn while resting. One should also be aware that extreme dieting without exercise and sufficient protein intake will result in the body consuming its own muscle mass, including the heart muscle. People who do not or cannot consume sufficient protein will essentially consume themselves until they die, if related diseases do not kill them first. So, consuming enough grams of protein each day is important (0.8 times your weight in kilograms, or about 0.36 times your weight in pounds). And each day you must do enough physical activity to keep your muscles from deteriorating.

How do you build muscle without the dreaded E-word? Incorporate muscle-building activity into your daily physical activity routine. For example, walking to your supermarket and carrying a bag or two of groceries back home will strengthen your legs, arms, back, and other muscles. Or digging a hole in your garden to plant a tree, instead of having a gardener do it for you, will build muscle and burn calories. Riding a bicycle also builds muscle and burns calories. Anything you can make yourself do physically is a help.

Whatever we do to burn more calories gets us closer to our weight loss goal. Even if we eat exactly the number of calories that we burned, the increased muscle mass will be burning a few more calories each day, while we rest and sleep, bringing us closer to our goals.

There are 3500 calories in a pound of fat. So, if you want to lose one pound, you must create a deficit of 3500 calories by eating less and/or burning more. Weight loss all boils down to this simple principle and is what the Calories3 spreadsheet is all about.

Suppose you want to lose two pounds per week. That is 2 * 3500 = 7000 calories per week deficit that must be created. It is that simple! Of course, such calories loss is surely easier said than done. That 7000 calories means we have to create a 1000 calorie *a day* deficit. Wow! That means that if we were eating 2500 calories per day, we must now reduce that to 1500 per day. But, by weighing what we eat and selecting foods prudently, we can easily achieve this.

Initially, you will be losing water that is tied up in the stored glycogen. Weight lost can be as much as 15 pounds or more *in a single week or two*. But, do not get full of yourself over this as it is only water. It takes about 2 weeks for this dominant water loss to end and for our weight loss to become, primarily, fat loss. Of course, you will be losing fat from the first day you begin a serious calorie reduction, but this will be masked by the water loss. After two weeks, a more meaningful Basal Metabolic Rate can be calculated, though this too will fluctuate according to your activity, eating, salt intake, and scale repeatability and accuracy. Do not be alarmed as this number changes on the Calories3 spreadsheet. This information is to give you an idea of what is going on in your body. For example, I "gained" 2 pounds yesterday, but can assure you that I did not eat an extra 7000 calories' worth of food. I ate some Chinese noodles and the carbohydrates and salt from the soy sauce caused at least 2 pounds of water retention. This will go away over the next couple of days, but such fluctuation is the sort of thing that adds variability to our extrapolated parameters, such as BMR, our time to goal, our weight by goal time, and any calorie adjustments that we should make.

This BMR is how many calories you had been consuming to *maintain* your weight. It will usually seem much higher than you thought because we unconsciously eat more and underestimate our portions. For this reason, it is paramount for you to buy a <u>digital scale that will read to at least a kilogram, with 1 gram accuracy</u>. Why not ounces and pounds? Most nutrition databases, such as the USDA's, (http://www.nal.usda.gov/fnic/foodcomp/search/) provide data in grams. If you must convert, know that there are approximately 2.2 lbs per kilogram, or 28 grams to an ounce. Although I am more comfortable with pounds and ounces, I record everything except my weight in grams, mainly because of this USDA database, which is exceptionally complete.

Accurately entering your weight each morning as well as your daily caloric intake lets the Calorie3 spreadsheet track your progress and make calculations based on these inputs, including letting you know what adjustments, if any, you need to make to achieve your goals. There *will* be adjustments because your body will slow your metabolism down as you reduce your caloric intake. Since your brain thinks it is starving and that food is scarce, evolution has led to our bodies slowing down to preserve calories when starving, and we do NOT want this when we *want* to lose weight. My resting heart rate was about 72 bpm when I started this weight loss, and a month later my heart rate had dropped to 60 bpm. That is a 20% reduction! That means that I am burning 20% fewer calories just sitting down and sleeping than I was before, and this must be considered in my calculations. This can be compensated, somewhat, by the dreaded E-word— exercise—and the building of muscle, but I have been lackadaisical in doing significant exercises. Also, as I lose weight, I am carrying less excess fat around, so my BMR will drop.

This can be discouraging to any dieter who, despite sticking to a diet, finds that the weight is not dropping as fast as it was earlier during dieting. C'est la vie. As we lose significant amounts of weight, our calorie deficit must be increased to maintain the same weight loss.

Again, note, that one should consult with his or her physician before undertaking any unusual exercise plan, eating plan, or any abrupt change to the level of physical activity.

8. Tracking Your Progress

Now, this is the fun part. This is where we implement the information in this book and enter our data into the Calories3 spreadsheet. Begin by entering the following inputs:

Starting Date (mo/da/yr):
Height (inches):
Present Weight (Lbs):
Goal Weight (Lbs):
Goal Date (mo/da/yr):

Be realistic with your goals—2 pounds per week or about 10 pounds of weight loss per month is considered *very aggressive* and is usually undertaken only under your physician's guidelines. This corresponds to 1000 calorie per day deficit, which is fine if you were consuming 4000 calories per day, but serious business if you were only consuming 2000 calories/day, which may not be possible to do if you were consuming less than 2000 calories per day. I have found my BMR initially to be about 3000 calories but now my BMR has already dropped to about 2200. So, to maintain my desired loss of 2 pounds per week, I can only eat 1200 calories per day—the 1000 calorie per day deficit. Thus, I have to pay close attention to my nutrition intake to make sure that I am eating properly. Eating at much below this calorie level becomes almost impossible to do and still get required nutrition. I take multi-vitamin and calcium supplements and I monitor my protein intake with the spreadsheet. **Again, consult your physician before undertaking a radical change in eating habits.**

Once you enter the above data, the Calories3 spreadsheet then calculates your Body Mass Index (BMI—not to be confused with BMR, which is the Basal Metabolic Rate), and your Goal BMI. Rather than absolute weight, physicians prefer to use BMI because it allows direct comparison of short people as well as tall people. A BMI of 18.5 to 25 is considered normal, 25-30 is overweight, and a BMI of over 30 is considered obese—the embarrassing O-word we prefer not to think about. You can read more about BMI at the Wikipedia page: http://en.wikipedia.org/wiki/Body_mass_index

A surprising number of people find themselves with a BMI well over 30... 35... and even 40. This is very unhealthy and is likely the reason you have bought this plan and are doing something once and for all to get your BMI below 25 and to keep it there. By the time you get your BMI there, you will find it easy to keep it there, but you will likely have to keep an eye on your weight forever.

Each day, enter your morning weight under the day of the week in column B. Under the weight heading, you have ten rows in which to enter the food you eat that day. Yes, this is a hassle for a busy person, but it is paramount to weigh your food and determine the calories, grams of protein, and carbohydrates. Enter that data into columns C, D, and E, respectively. (Column C, in the yellow highlighted row, will display your totals for that day. Column F will show your average caloric intake, and column G will display your current BMI. The remaining columns will not be filled in until two weeks go by.)

On the 15th day, your Basal Metabolic Rate (BMR) will be calculated each day, along with your average weight loss per week, your expected weight at this rate by your goal date, and any adjustment necessary to keep on track. Thus, if you keep on track, you can predict your weight at any given time in the future. This adjustment column, K, is the number of calories you must add to (black) or subtract from (red) your daily intake to keep on track. Columns L and up are for your own notes, and if you are adept with Excel®, you can add your own cells and calculations. For example, if I make a dish like salmon chowder, I record all the ingredients:

	Salmon Corn Chowder			
corn	720	16	160	
carrrots	200	4	43	
potatoes	800	21	181	
salmon	720	107	0	
skim milk	550	53	80	
Onion(300g)	120	3	28	
1.5 gal	**3110**	**204**	**492**	17 svgs
13 oz bowl	183	12	29	serving
11oz Cup	156	10	25	

I let Excel® total the columns and perform the math to determine the number of servings and the calories, grams protein, and grams carbs per serving. Similarly, if I make a loaf of bread, I will weigh each of the ingredients, enter their calories, sum them all, then weigh the completed loaf. That contains the total number of calories, the total grams of protein, and the total grams of carbohydrate, so I then know how much of what it is per 100 grams, and so on. It is an area where YOU can add notes or calculations.

Our weight is dependent on so many factors, like salt intake the day before, carbohydrate intake the day before, the fiber intake the day before, whether or not you have had a bowel movement recently, how much exercise you have done, whether you built up any muscle, and the accuracy and repeatability of your scale. So, this adjustment number—even though it is somewhat smoothed by averaging over the preceding two weeks-- is not to be taken *too* seriously. But, if it continually shows in the red, then it is an indicator that you must reduce your daily calorie intake slightly, increase your daily activity slightly, or set a more realistic goal. Ideally, you keep the adjustment calories in column K as close to zero as possible.

The following are examples of a couple of typical days:

Day#	FOOD ITEM	Calories	Protein(g)	Carb(g)	Av Cal/Day	BMI	BMR	lb/wk	Avg. Wt. By Goal Date	Adjust Cal/day
34	Saturday, August 20, 2011	1517	97	147	1195	39.5	2525	2.9	231	245
	Wt.(Lbs): 267.4									
	skim milk powder & 35g Whey Protein	180	37	8						
	Fruit Salad(400g)	175	6	42						
	Cottage Cheese(2%)(140g)	120	17	5						
	Beer	150	2	13						
	Eggs(2)	140	13	1						
	Potato(85g)	60	2	14						
	Cherries (50g)	32	0	8						
	Chinese food	300	20	40						
	Wine(15oz)	360	0	16						
35	Sunday, August 21, 2011	1470	135	130	1203	39.3	2703	3.4	230	292
	Wt.(Lbs): 266.0									
	skim milk powder & 35g Whey Protein	180	37	8						
	Fruit Salad(400g)	175	6	42						
	Cottage Cheese(2%)(200g)	175	24	7						
	Carrots(295g)	120	3	28						
	2 cans V-8	140	6	30						
	Coors Light (1 can)	100	1	6						
	Chicken Leg (170g)+Chicken Wing(50g)	535	56	0						
	Summer Squash(220g)	45	2	9						
36	Monday, August 22, 2011	1470	125	161	1211	39.7	2229	1.4	239	(157)
	Wt.(Lbs): 268.6									
	skim milk powder & 35g Whey Protein	180	37	8						
	Oatmeal (350g)	325	13	58						
	Nutri(20g)	115	3	7						
	Fruit Salad(350g)	155	4	37						
	Salmon Chowder (13oz)	185	12	29						
	Salad(275)	100	5	22						
	chicken breast(200g) w/o skin	410	51	0						

You may have to zoom in to read the above data, but I want to make a few points about it. First, you will notice the changing BMR, Wt. By Goal Date, and Adjust Cal/day columns. The reason for this is because on the 36th day, the weight actually went *up* by more than two pounds due, most likely, to the salt in the Chinese food and carbohydrates in the wine and beer on the 34th and 35th days. This caused the adjustment to jump from a surplus of 245 calories/day, to a surplus of 292 calories/day, then down to a deficit of 157 calories/day. The surplus means one should eat MORE calories than they have been eating and the deficit (red) means they need to cut back a bit more. These are smoothed averages over the preceding two weeks, so they are *rough* indicators as to what adjustments a person needs to make to his or her calorie intake.

So, those extrapolated columns have a lot of "noise" in them and should be viewed only as trends. In other words, if the Adjust calorie/day column is consistently red, you would want to reduce your calories by the approximate amount shown until it occasionally shows a black, positive, number. The idea is to keep this as near to zero as possible, which will be an indication that you are exactly on track to reach your goal.

Another question I would like to answer is what to do if you run out of rows. You simply combine the rows as I do in my example with the skim milk powder and 35 grams of whey protein, especially since I have that daily. I use the skim milk powder in my coffee as a creamer, and I either have the scoop of whey protein with my fruit and cottage cheese or later in the day with a suitable food, like the chowder. Either way, I consume that combination daily.

While you *could* look up the calories for each dish daily on the USDA chart, it is sometimes easier to use a calculator and ratio it from previous days. For example, if one day I eat 200g of cottage cheese and only 100g of the cottage cheese the next day, I can simply enter half the calories, half the protein, and half the carbohydrates of the previous day's cottage cheese consumption, and so on. The whole point is for you to get used to eating your target amounts and to learn what foods have what combinations of calories, protein, and carbohydrates for a given serving. One of the first snacks I had was celery with a "little" peanut butter. Ha! I later realized that the "little" peanut butter was 300 calories! I am very careful with calorie-laden foods like peanut butter now. Contrast that with zucchini, of which I can eat a pound and only ingest 77 calories, with 5 grams protein and 16 grams carbohydrate. Yesterday, I had a chicken leg and wing, which had an astonishing 535 calories, thus putting me over my quota for the second day in a row. I am careful to be under quota today and in the days ahead to get back on track. These red numbers will haunt me for a while. I will also increase my exercise level to get my weight back on track.

Thus, as we continue down the road of weighing our food and learning foods' calories, protein, and carbohydrate contents, if/when we go to a restaurant or eat in someone's home, we can eyeball the approximate amounts of each food and make a reasonable "guestimate". Then when we get home and record what we have eaten. We also know which foods to avoid and which foods to minimize. Recently, I was served a steak, twice-baked potato, green beans, and garlic bread. I ate all the foods, but took half my steak and half (of a half) potato home with me, and only ate the smallest piece of garlic bread, which I estimated to be 250 calories with the generous amount of butter on it. I looked up the foods on the USDA database and entered my best guess as to the quantity I had consumed. I ultimately made 3 meals out of that piece of steak, each with about 250 calories.

I have ordered a small pocket/purse sized scale for keeping myself honest when eating out. The one I chose was only $5 from Amazon.com and is described as: Electronic Digital Weighting Pocket Scale 0.1g-1000g. With a range of 1000g (2.2 lbs) I can set my plate on it, note the weight, then remove a piece of meat or potato and note the difference. Most digital scales let you press the TARE button which zeros the scale with whatever is placed upon it. Since negative weights do not make sense, *removing* a piece of food from the plate will result in a readout of the weight of that food. Going to such an extreme to weigh food in restaurants is pretty obsessive, I will admit, but the more accuracy I put into the Calories3 spreadsheet, the better the accuracy of its predictions will be.

9. Final Notes

The techniques described here of weighing one's food, looking up and calculating calories/protein/carbohydrate grams, then entering the data into the Calories3 spreadsheet is a royal pain in the butt, make no mistake about it. But mastering the Calories3 spreadsheet can be fun and you will see progress soon. Moreover, this method is foolproof. If you accurately enter your calories and your weight, the calculated parameters will be as accurate as possible, as will the predictions. You will also find it exciting to watch your progress. You will understand where the excess calories were coming from and learn how to combat that tendency in the future.

Most important for me is to watch my carbohydrate intake so that I do not stimulate my over-active appetite and can keep it under control. Everyone knows what a drag it is to be hungry, so eating foods to minimize that hunger is paramount for me, otherwise my willpower can be overloaded. I am also amazed at what I used to eat in the past, thinking erroneously that it was only a couple of hundred calories, when it was several times that much, mainly baked goods like bread. I could easily eat 500 calories or more just in bread, waiting hungrily for a restaurant meal to be served. Salads, by themselves, are nutritious and very low in calories, but if I add cheese, croutons, and salad dressing to the salad, the calories skyrocket! **A Caesar salad can contain more calories than a cheeseburger!!!**

Also worth mentioning is that like the watched pot that takes forever to boil, losing weight takes forever to lose. Even an aggressive 2.2 pounds per week is less than a third of a pound per day, below the accuracy and repeatability of most bathroom scales. So, one can see a couple of days or more without ANY apparent progress and that can be discouraging.

But, you know what you are eating and if you are eating less than your BMR, you are losing weight. Period! Even if your scale fails to show weight loss for a few days, you are losing weight. You may have absorbed excess water due to salt intake or your menstrual cycle. This is not fat and is temporary. Drinking plenty of water is important—10 to12 glasses/day—to make sure you can flush out excess salt. It is counter-intuitive to drink water to lose water, but salt makes us retain water and drinking water will help flush out the salt.

So, don't sweat the small variations in your weight loss. Just keep on with your plan and eat accordingly to reach your goal, and you most certainly will. You might need adjustments along the way, but that will be either from the fact that you are reducing your BMR by losing weight or insufficiently exercising. In either case, a reduction in calorie intake may be required, but the Calories3 spreadsheet will guide you.

I am confidently writing this book before even reaching my goals, but I can do so because this is **FOOLPROOF**. People can try all sorts of exotic diets and achieve varying results, but this diet lets you eat anything you wish, if you are prepared for the consequences. You will still lose weight if you eat a burger and fries, but that may be ALL that you can eat the entire day, and you will be famished with your blood sugar cycling extremely. I would rather eat a healthy breakfast with fruit and cottage cheese, choose a snack for lunch, and have a steak or fish or chicken and vegetables for dinner. You may prefer to eat ham and eggs for breakfast and salads for lunch and dinner. If you do that, beware that salad dressing is largely made from oil—fat. Caesar salad, for example, can have much more than 500 grams of fat in it—it is not a diet food.

This is an exciting learning experience for you! You will be learning the details of what your body has been trying to tell you, and you will learn the details of the calorie, protein, and carbohydrate content of the foods you enjoy. You will experience shocks from how many calories some of your favorite goodies contain. You are also in for some pleasant surprises as you learn that you can eat some foods as much as you want—with impunity.

Today is an exciting time for you in that you know you have a plan. **This is it!** This is the plan that will let you achieve your goal! You will never have to say, "I tried the such-and-so diet and it didn't work." This diet cannot fail because it is not a "diet"—it is an eating plan that YOU choose, around the foods that YOU like, albeit not likely in the *quantities* that you like. It is an eating plan with detailed feedback so you know and understand the consequences of **your** decisions. The only way that you will not lose weight is if you choose not to follow your plan. But, if you follow your plan, guided by this book and the Calories3 spreadsheet, you WILL achieve your goal in a healthy way, and you will keep it off with your new-found knowledge.

Be sure to visit http://WeightAgency.com for additional information, products, and support. Share your success stories by emailing me at bobbie@weightagency.com.

www.ingramcontent.com/pod-product-compliance
Lightning Source LLC
Chambersburg PA
CBHW070239290526
45789CB00004B/1692